Traditional Body Care Methods

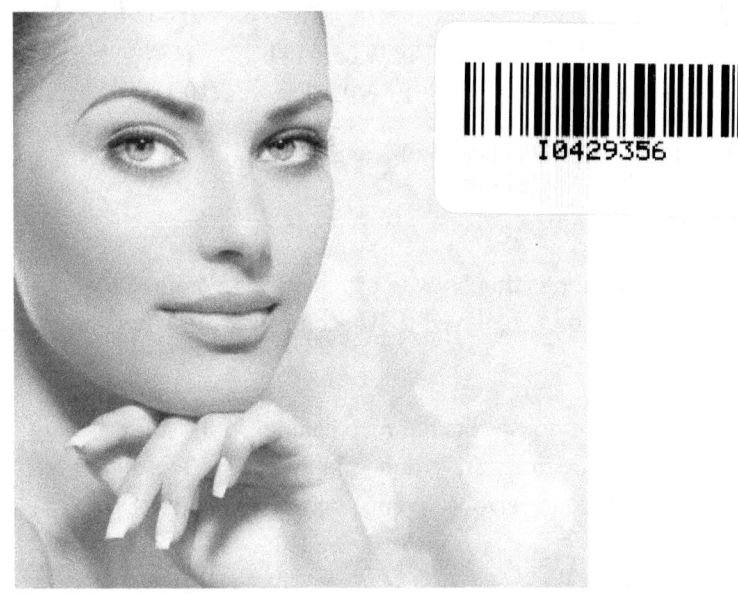

Natural Ancient Ways to Keep Your Body, Hands, and Feet Beautiful and Younger Looking

Dueep Jyot Singh

Mendon Cottage Books

Health Learning Series

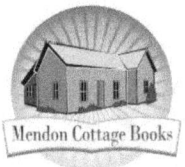

JD-Biz Publishing

Download Free Books!

http://MendonCottageBooks.com

Our books are available at

1. Amazon.com

2. Barnes and Noble

3. Itunes

4. Kobo

5. Smashwords

6. Google Play Books

Download Free Books!

http://MendonCottageBooks.com

Table of Contents

Introduction

I was reading one of my favorite authors, Rex Stout, and Archie Goodwin, my favorite narrator spoke about one of their clients who he did not like. She was loudmouthed, rude, overdressed, and he was glad to see that he had an excuse not to like her. She had an unwashed neck.

I gave a grin of smug and superior pomposity. Washing behind my ears, and washing my neck properly every day when having a bath had been drilled into me when I was a baby. So I had a squeaky clean neck, hurray, hurray. But it looked like I had been neglecting my elbows and my knees and also my feet. That comes of having no time for leisurely showers because one is in too much of a hurry to shower, get ready, and get out of the house in time to catch the morning's rush to the rat race.

Even if you are not rushing around, and you have all the time in the world to have a long leisurely bath with all those lotions, potions, bath salts, and all those chemical-based stuffs, let us look at natural methods which are going to add to a clean body and exterior.

These notions of elementary hygiene and cleanliness were disregarded, in many parts of the world, especially in Europe for centuries, but in other parts of the world, especially in ancient civilizations like Egypt, Persia, Babylon, China, Japan, and even ancient Europe, traditional beauty recipes to take care of the body and keep it young, youthful looking, and beautiful were handed down from grandmother to grandchild, and utilized.

Nowadays, so many of us are so busy buying really expensive brand name cosmetics, and slathering them all over our skins, that we have forgotten all about natural-based traditional methods which have been in use for millenniums, especially in body and hand care.

People always admire beautiful and well-maintained hands because they are about as expressive and appealing a feature to enhance your personality as a beautifully formed and made up youthful looking face is.

The time spent upon taking care of your hands, feet, and the rest of your body can never be thought wasted. However, hands and feet and other parts of your body only get a fraction of the care and attention, we lavish upon our faces.

If you think that a hand is not expressive look at the soft and smooth, graceful gestures of a dancer using both her hands to express a variety and gamut of emotions. It is sheer poetry and you may often have seen women using their hands so gracefully even in normal day-to-day gestures. This may make you feel so envious.

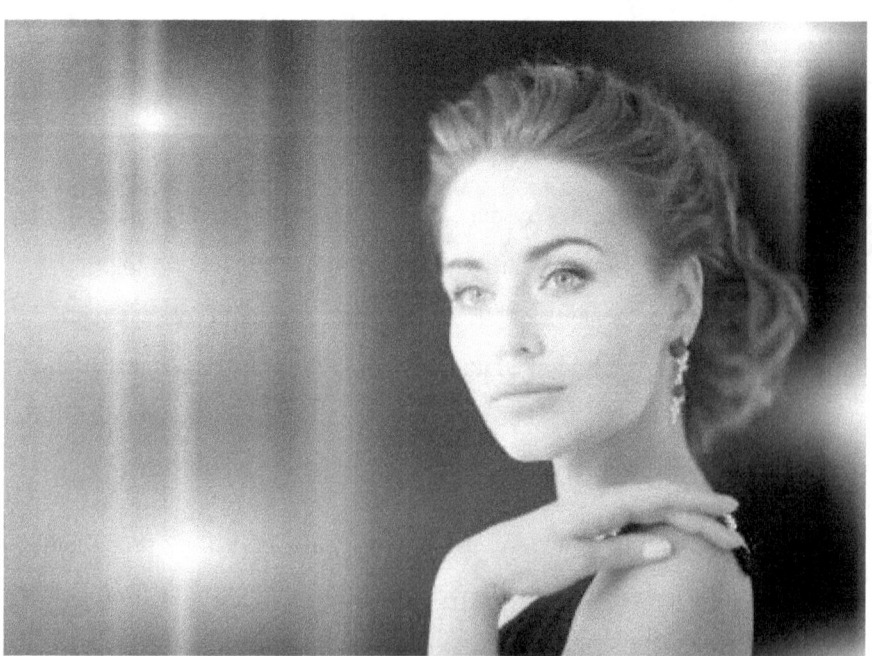

Being quite human ourselves, we look at the ill cared for, rough skinned, and possibly red hands and decided that we are going to do something about it tomorrow.

Well, tomorrow is here today, and this book is going to tell you all about traditional recipes made from items found right there in your kitchen, and in any traditional kitchen, with natural products.

Skin Cleansing Rubs

In ancient times, the skin was kept clean by excoriating the skin surface with a natural rub. In the East, a dry powder material base was used in which a liquid was put. In Europe, oatmeal and bran was used as a powdery base. In other parts of the world, you could use chickpea powder. All of these are healthy materials and totally natural, and have been long used for skin cleansers.

For Oily Skin

For this you are going to use an oatmeal scrub. Traditionally, especially in Asia, these scrubs were taken in the bathing area, where one did not bother much if the ground was stained with oil and turmeric. Turmeric is a spice used often in cooking in Asia. For millenniums, it has also been used as a beauty product to protect the skin from disease, keep it youthful looking, glowing, and getting rid of blemishes and other skin ailments.

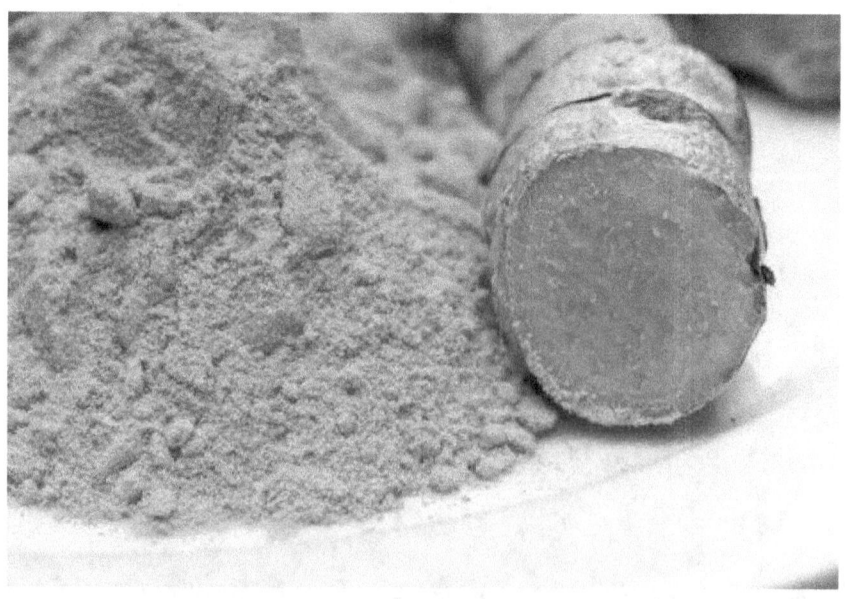

Remember that turmeric is capable of staining clothes and skin. So if you use this in a beauty preparation made by you, get rid of all vestiges of turmeric by cleaning the surface with a cotton wad dipped in milk or yogurt.

To make a bath scrub you are going to take 60 g – 15 tablespoons – of chickpea powder/oatmeal powder/bran/and half a spoonful of turmeric. Now you are going to add a little bit of milk to it, so that you do not have to bother about staining.

This is going to be your cleansing agent and soap from now on to keep your skin disease free. To this, you can add 1 tablespoon full of your favorite oil to moisturize the skin, like olive oil, sesame oil, I use coconut oil, and beat it until you get a thick paste.

This is what you are going to use on your face, neck, arms, hands, feet, elbows, and knees. That means you are ready for your shower in your bathroom, and uncluttered with clothing.

Now sit in your bathroom, bring a book with you to read It is going to take anywhere between 10 to 15 minutes for this mixture to start to dry up on the surface of the skin. In ancient times, women used to do this treatment in their women's baths, especially in Turkish hamams where they had slaves and eunuchs to do the rubbing and scrubbing and massaging of those spoilt little butterflies.

But you are going to be doing the rubbing and scrubbing yourself with the palms of your hands.

You will be surprised to see the amount of dirt coming off in small dry scrubbed pieces of paste. I tried this experiment on myself once. I cleaned my face with some cleansing lotion borrowed from a colleague – I do not use chemical-based makeup – and after that, I washed my face with cleansing soap, and hot water.

After that, I thought my skin was quite clean, but I wanted to see what this cleansing traditional method would do to a skin which was already clean.

The answer was that your skin can never be too clean. I was astonished at the particles of dust, coming off, not exactly as grime, – thanks to the soap and water and chemical-based cleanser – but still as gray external layers of skin.

This last cleansing was done due to the milk. So remember that milk is the best natural cleanser available to mankind today.

Remember to have a bath with warm water. This is going to get rid of any vestiges of turmeric stain. This natural antiseptic is excellent to give you a young and youthful look.

Scrub well with your loofah to get the blood circulation moving.

A loofah is the interior fiber of the ridge gourd.

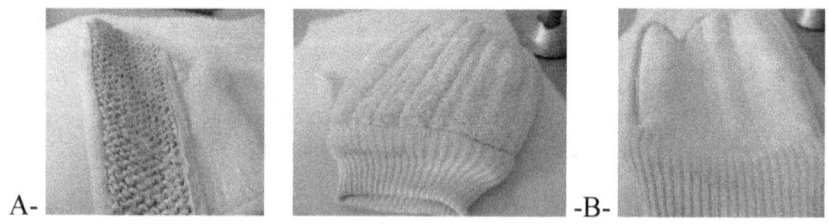

Sisal and loofah gourd gloves - 2 designs

Nowadays, you can get this as a hand glove for scrubbing with the loofah on one side and cotton fabric on the other side.[1] (B)

Nevertheless, I managed to get my hundred percent natural loofah by borrowing it from a gardener friend who had plenty of ridge gourds growing in his garden. I picked a large one, and put it in the sun. After that I removed the dry outer covering, 3 – 4 days sunning would crack it – I got rid of all the seeds inside the plant, planted some in my garden, and allowed my loofah to dry.

For centuries, this has been the best way in which you scrub yourself and get your circulation moving after a bath. That is, of course, after you have scrub yourself with a skin rub to get rid of the blemishes, skin patches, wrinkles, and darkness of the skin.

Also, turmeric is the best depilatory which has been used for centuries. One fine day, when I was putting on my sports clothes at college, I noticed that the rest of the team members had really hairy arms and even legs. There was something wrong with me, because my arms and legs did not have any hair at all, I thought. Not a single hair.

The reason was that when I was a baby my grandmother used to rub my skin with a paste made up of mustard oil, turmeric, and chickpea to clean her little baby's skin before I was allowed to bake in the sun, so that my muscles would grow normally, and strong. This was the only time when children of our times were allowed to play in the dirt before we reached school age.

---

[1] http://www.ebay.com/itm/LOOFAH-EXFOLIATOR-GLOVE-sisal-lufah-bath-mitt-shower-mitten-/161980499902?hash=item25b6ca47be:g:9CIAAOSwe7BWxD7q

Nowadays, for a number of parents, the idea of their children playing in the dirt is going to sound horrible and abhorrent, but they do not know that children need to have lots of fresh air, exposure to the sun, and the elements and also to the dirt so that they build up a natural resistance to organisms in the dirt through continuous exposure to them.

So we fell down in the mud and got thoroughly dusty and had the most enjoyable time of our lives. This exercise also helped our muscles to grow properly.

When we began going to school, this massage was done over the weekends, or in the evening, if grandma had the energy or inclination or saw one little hair growing anywhere on our legs or hands. The playing in the mud continued, of course, in our own gardens. We never came inside the house unless absolutely necessary or at lunchtime and to go to sleep.

After 3 hours, I would be given a warm water bath – in a little pink possibly plastic bathtub, which alas did not last more than 3 generations – scrubbed thoroughly with a rough piece of fabric, and then imprisoned in my pram or popped into my crib.

Even today, my hands and legs are completely hairless, thanks to the turmeric and oil/bran/chickpea scrub done when I was a baby. The same thing goes for youngsters my age and of my generation who had traditional grandmas to take care of them. Even today, you can see this baking in the sun, after an oil massage being done for children and adults in many parts of the world because of its healthy natural benefits.

So how and when to use this rub?

You are going to use it half an hour before you have your bath or you can do it before you go to sleep, half an hour before you sleep, and then take your late-night shower and then pop into bed. This is a good option for all those people who do not have the time to have a shower, first thing in the morning before they go off to their office in a hurry.

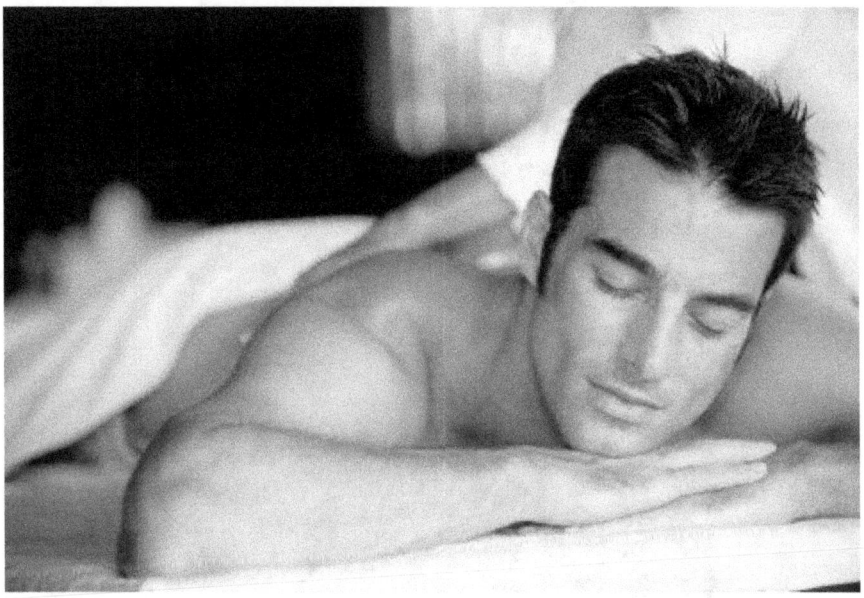

Massage, especially on tissue which has been injured, as a therapeutic remedy or just for relaxation has been en vogue for centuries.

Do this in the initial stages, continuously, once a day for the first 3 days. After that, you can do it every second and third day, because your skin has already begun to grow clean and expects this natural treatment instead of chemical-based soap and water.

Do this, 6 times at an interval of 2 – 3 days. After that, you can do it once every week. In the winter, do this once every 2 weeks, depending on how cold it is.

You are going to find a distinct change in your skin texture and color tone, within 6 – 7 rubs. That is because of the turmeric.

Since ancient times, turmeric and milk have been used as a way in which one's skin tone was made lighter, especially in areas where there was plenty of sun.

Incidentally, if this treatment is done to a child on the face when young, he is never going to suffer from acne and skin problems when he hits his teens.

Skin Blemishes

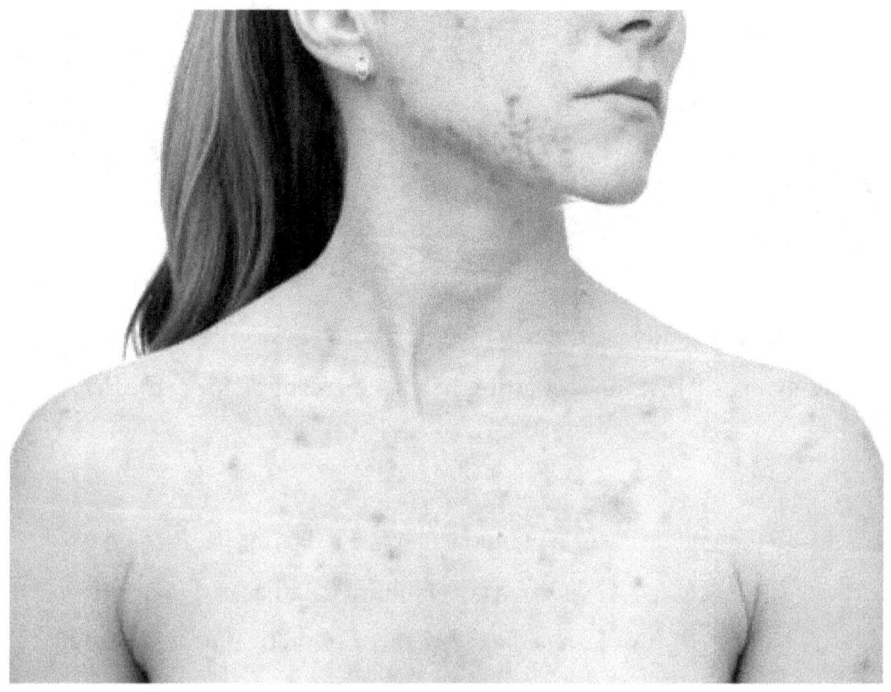

In ancient Scandinavia, the Norse beauties kept their skin beautiful, young, and youthful looking, with just one traditional natural recipe. Before they went to sleep, they scrubbed their faces with a mixture made up of milk cream and salt.

Salt is the best exfoliator. The cream is the moisturizer. Along with that, they used bran in which they added milk as a cleanser. Like I said before, oatmeal, bran, and any other powdered cereal can be used as a base, depending on where you are on the earth, and you are going to have local traditional beauty enhancing recipes with that cereal – wheat flour, bran, chickpea, oatmeal, and other grains – have been used for millenniums.

If you want to remove blemishes on your skin, you can use warm milk. In fact, I regret not doing this treatment during this winter, because the weather was too cold and I was too lazy and according to me, now that spring is here, my skin looks dull, lifeless, and absolutely without a glow. Give me 2 days, and milk cream with a little bit of lemon and some salt in it. I am going to do this treatment, 3 times a day over the next weekend when I do not intend going out in the sun. The milk has to be warm. I may add a little bit of honey to it, because I just like honey!

In ancient times, the milk was taken fresh from the cow, goat, sheep, or any other source of milk – including camels, yaks, and other domesticated animals, and used straight on the skin, including foaming milk applied either by the fingertips and massaged into the skin until all of the milk has been absorbed and left on for 20 minutes; or left on without any massaging and then washed with fresh cold water in the summer and warm water in the winter is the best beauty treatment, you can give your body.

Remember that you are not going to use any soap with this treatment. The problem with chemical-based soaps is that people have become so used to being told that their skins cannot do without them, that they begin to believe that.

If you think that there is some sort of stickiness brought on by the oil after you have a shower, do not remove it with soap and water. Instead, have a paste of one part of chickpea powder/oatmeal powder/wheat flour/and 2 parts of milk all over your body and scrub off all the oil, which will get absorbed in the cereal.

So you may want to ask me what I use upon my face and for body care and I have been using traditionally, – when I do not use makeup, or powder or moisturizers or lotions or cleansers or any of that stuff, but still have a young and youthful looking skin?

That is easy. One spoonful of natural cold cream taken off milk, right from the fridge, to this I add just this little pinch of turmeric. This is my soap, cleanser, moisturizer, lotion, and any skin care treatment, used every day. I have never suffered from dry skin, even though I may go out in freezing temperatures, especially in the winter. Nor through dehydrated skin, chapped skin, or any sort of skin infection ever.

Combination Skins

This means that some areas are going to be dry and some areas are going to be oily. For this, you are going to use a traditional art known as Fuller's earth.

When I was at college, all my seniors used to use this instead of soap. That is because they had been taught since childhood, that this was the best way in which they could get rid of the open pores in their skin and leave it smooth, silky, clean, and without any blemish.

You are going to put 4 tablespoons full of Fuller's Earth[2] in a cup full of water, and make a paste of it. If it is in solid form, it is going to take 2 hours for it to become enough of a paste without any lumps. Depending on your physique, you will have to estimate the amount of powder needed to cover your face, and the rest of your body.

Apply it all over your face and body, and sit in the shade for just half an hour, soaking up the sun in the summer. In the winter, you are going to sit in the winter sun like the ancients did.

You are going to take a warm water bath in the winter after half an hour. In winter, you can take a cold water or fresh water bath. This soaking of the sun is to get rid of the oil content on your skin.

You are going to find all the dirt removed from the surface of the skin, and tone of your skin, while lightening your complexion.

If your skin is dry or oily, you do not need to worry about when and how to use Fuller's Earth. You are going to use it once a week. So if you think your skin feels dry and lifeless, get the life back into it along with its natural softness with this natural Earth.

Remember that true original Fuller's Earth is always going to be light yellow – cream in color. If you have any Fuller Earth clods with hints of rust color/Brown, Do Not Use It. Those are impurities in the pure earth. Possibly dead fossils and other minerals present in those pieces of natural earth.

---

[2]

http://www.ebay.com/sch/i.html?_from=R40&_trksid=p2050601.m570.l1313.TR3.TRC2.A0.H0.XMultani+mitti.TRS0&_nkw=Multani+mitti&_sacat=0

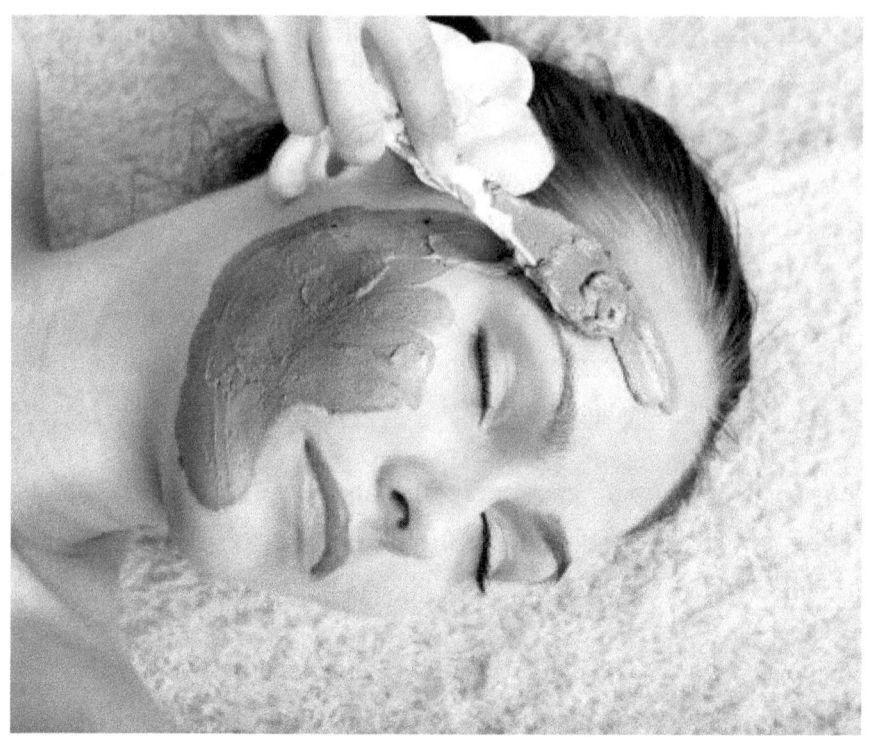

This is the treatment, which you is being done in those expensive spas. The base is Fuller's Earth, with a number of ingredients including milk and honey, being added to the mixture, along with other sweet smelling natural herbs like possibly sandalwood powder. And one spa treatment sets you back anywhere between $450 – $500 for ingredients which should not cost you more than a total of $25 which will give you enough of material for 25 spa treatments. Do the math.

Dull and Lifeless Hair

One of my friends kept complaining that her hair was absolutely dull and lifeless and she could do nothing with it. So I told her that I had an expensive paste which I had got from abroad, and it was really, really expensive. I emphasized the expensive part a lot. After demurring a bit, whether I really wanted to give her any of my precious mixture, because who knew when I would go to the USA again, and all that jazz, I managed to persuade myself to part with this solution, being so altruistic but I would bring it to the office myself. But she had to follow the instructions very carefully.

Call me a bit of a ham, but then, the first rule of marketing, which I taught to my students as a marketing instructor, at that time was the more showmanship you put into your selling and the more demand you create for an object, the more they will want it, price no concern. That is the theory on what multibillion-dollar brand names are existing.

When I came back in the evening, I powdered some Fuller's Earth and filtered it. To this I added some rose petals just for show. Along with some powdered sandalwood powder. Just for the fragrance. And I knew she was going to take a hearty sniff, when I handed her this mixture. So if it smelled expensive, it had to be expensive.

I mixed them all together and told her that when she went home, she was going to make a paste of this powder with a little bit of warm water, *"remember warm water or shall I write it down for you, S and she nodding her head very impressed – all patter and showmanship"* – and spread that paste all over your scalp, and on your hair.

Leave it on for half an hour, and then wash your hair with warm water – and nothing else to get rid of all the paste. This is going to get rid of all the dandruff, and keep your hair, silky, manageable, and within control.

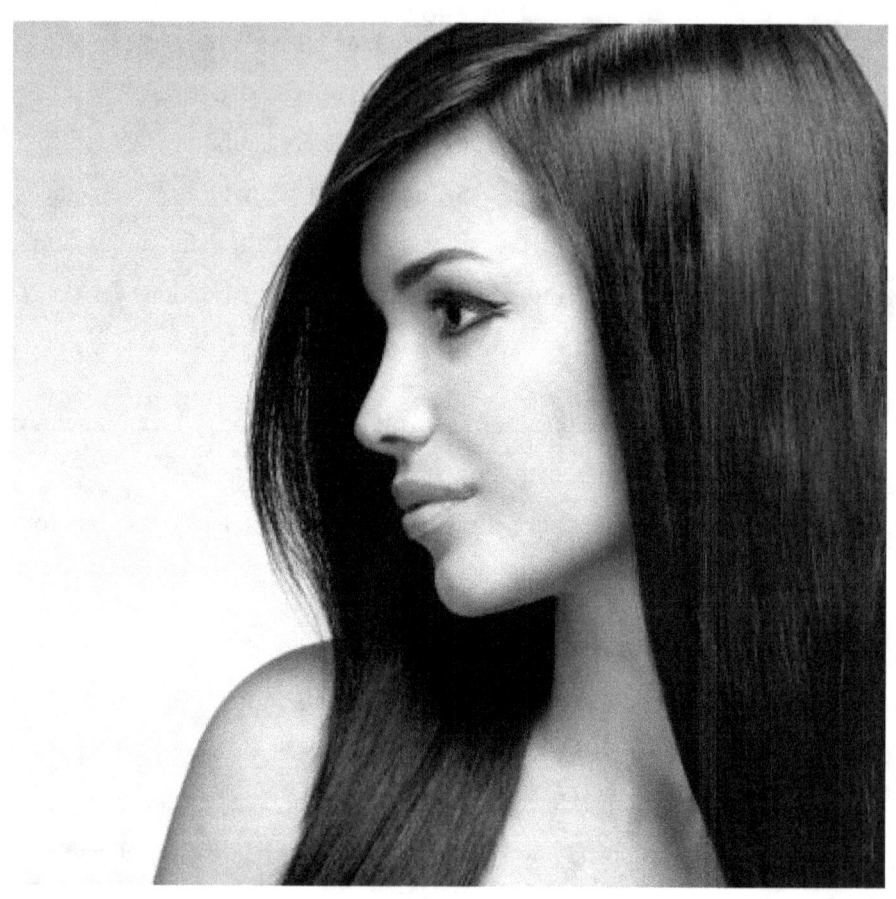

The only problem was the results were so good that every week, she wanted this mixture with which to wash her hair. And I could not sell her something; price no concern – as coming directly from abroad – because I am not at all business minded at that time. And also I did not want to get into the responsibility of keeping her supplied with this powder every week.

So I had to pretend that my mixture was finished and sorry I was not going back to the USA anytime soon to replenish my stock of natural expensive hair managing powder. She stopped talking to me, because what sort of friend was I, I could not do this little thing for her? Sulk, sulk.

A decade has passed since then and I do not know where she is today but this is for the rest of my friends out there. Who cannot manage their hair and want them to be squeaky clean, long, silky, without resort to chemical-based shampoos.

Problems of Excessive Sweating

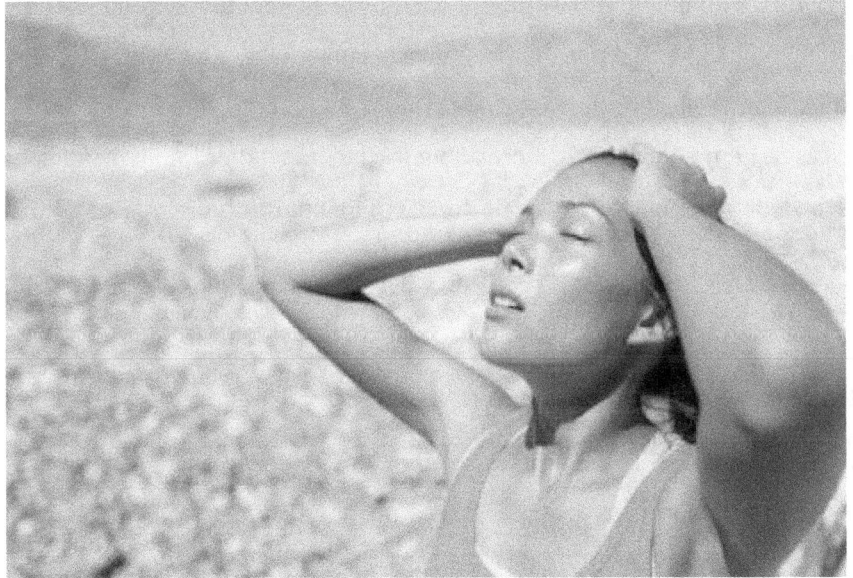

An extremely foolish action without any head covering and skin being exposed directly to the sun without protective clothing on the body.

During my life full of extensive travel, I have been in many climates, and I have found that in many parts of the world, especially in tropical areas, they had their natural ways of protecting themselves from the sun, especially during the summer. One was of course not coming out in the sun from 11 to 4 except if absolutely necessary, and never in the midday sun.

Even then, many people suffered from excessive sweating, especially when sometimes the sweat stunk and left behind an unpleasant yellow stain on their cotton garments.

Hyperhidrosis And Mud Therapy

Believe it or not, mud therapy to cure a number of diseases naturally has been used throughout the world, for ages since ancient times. A number of natural muds like Red Sea mud in Jordan, ordinary River mud in Africa, and Fuller's Earth have been in use for centuries, in order to cure a number of diseases. I am going to talk more about mud therapy after I tell you all about excessive sweating, which can be cured with a mud bath.

Hyperhidrosis is an age-old problem, where you are going to find yourself sweating excessively the moment you go into a temperature zone above room temperature.

In ancient times, mud therapy was used to cure this problem. The body was slathered with soft mud the procedure which I am going to tell you right now.

Mud therapy is one of the most effective, beneficial, and simple treatment known to man. The mud which is used for this therapy is lump free, clean, and taken from 3 – 4 feet depth from the surface of the ground so that it does not have any sort of organic contamination, pieces of rock, or chemical manures in it.

Mud is one of the 5 natural elements found in nature, and that is why it has an immense impact on your body, while you are well, also while you are ill.

Benefits of Using Mud

The effects of mud are naturally invigorating, revitalizing, and refreshing. For skin diseases and wounds, in ancient times, mud therapy was the only true bandage, with mud taken straight from a healthy water source, the wound or affected area washed properly, cleaned, and the mud applied directly on the injured skin.

This supposedly according to the ancients drew away all the poisons. Also, mud therapy diluted and absorbed the toxic substances in the body and ultimately eliminated them.

Mud was used in ancient times successfully in different diseases like constipation, headache, skin diseases, and even high blood pressure.

Here are some more advantages of using natural mud –

The color is supposed to absorb all the beneficial colors of the sun and convey them to the body.

Mud is going to retain moisture for a long time when it is applied over the body. Also, it cools down the surface temperature of the skin. That is why in ancient times, when patients suffered from fever, they were immediately slathered with a mud solution, so that the water in the mud along with its natural healing ingredients could be used to cool the temperature, as well as heal the body naturally.

The best thing about mud is that its consistency and shape can be changed easily by adding as much water as necessary.

Best of all, mud is cheap, and easily available all over the world. You may find areas where special mud is taken especially from lakes in Europe, and from the Red Sea and so on. This mud is going to be dried, powdered, and sieved so that you can remove stones, grass particles, and extraneous material as well as other impurities, especially if it has been taken from the bottom of the sea, to get pure helpful mud.

Local Application of Mud

If you have not tried out a little bit of mud therapy, you may be tempted to try it out this weekend.

Try it out in the initial stages on your stomach, your torso, hands, and legs – just as an experiment to get rid of stomach problems and to see the visible effect on the body with a little bit of pampering with mud.

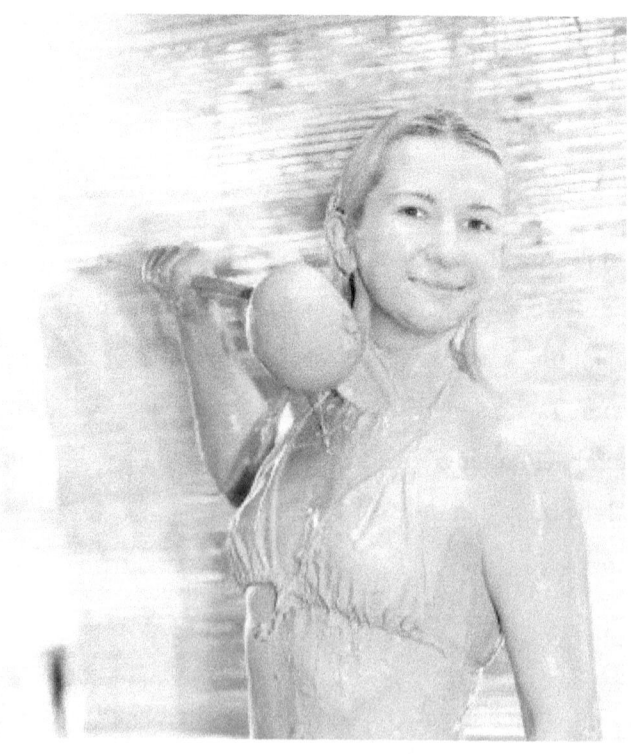

You are going to spread the soaked mud onto a thin, wet muslin cloth. Apply it in a thin and flat layer, depending on the area which you are going to cover. The duration of a mud pack application is going to be 20 – 30 minutes. When you are applying it in the winter, you can place a blanket over the mud pack and cover the body as well, to prevent it from being exposed to the cold.

Benefits of Mud Packs

Apart from cooling down the skin, it relieves you from every form of indigestion, especially when it is applied on the abdominal area. It is effective in decreasing intestinal heat, and also stimulates the digestive system to work properly and naturally.

A thick mud pack, applied on your head is going to get rid of chronic and congestive headaches. In ancient times, people suffering from headaches just went to the nearest mud source, – River Tigris, River Nile, – scooped up handfuls of mud, from under the bottom surface, and applied it all over the aching area.

After that they went home knowing that the pain would be soon gone with the wind. So if you are suffering from a chronic, congestive headache, try this treatment out by applying any black mud, or fuller's earth, on that area.

In ancient times, applying mud packs over the eyes was helpful in cases of conjunctivitis, itching, errors of refraction like short sightedness and long sightedness and also in glaucoma where it helped to reduce tension in the eyeball.

A mud pack for the face was done by soaking mud and applying the paste all over the face. This was then allowed to dry for 30 minutes. This was helpful in improving the complexion of the skin and removing pimples. It also opened the skin pores and eliminated toxins from the surface of the skin. This was also helpful in eliminating dark circles around the eyes.

The face was washed thoroughly with cold water to close up the pores, after half an hour when the mud pack was rubbed off with a little bit of warm water to get rid of the dead cells. After the surface was clean of mud, it was scrubbed well with cold water.

Black circles and wrinkles are thus going to be removed with periodic applications of mud packs.

Having a Mud Bath

You are going to apply mud on yourself with you either sitting down or lying down. This is going to help to improve the skin condition by increasing the circulation and also energizing the skin tissues.

Care should be taken to avoid catching any sort of cold during this bath. Afterwards, you should take a cold shower with a strong jet spray. You can also use a warm jet spray, depending on the temperature.

You are then going to dry yourself quickly and pop inside a warm bed.

A mud bath duration can be anywhere between 40 – 60 minutes, depending on how effective you want the treatment to be.

So now, let us continue on with how you are going to get rid of the problem of excessive sweating by applying a paste of fuller's earth all over the body. This is also an excellent cure for prickly heat, especially in the summer.

Also, if you are suffering from hyperhidrosis, cut out the salt intake. You are going to find an immediate and visible beneficial effect.

In ancient times, Eastern beauties kept their skin cool, younger looking, acne free, blackhead free, blemish free, and spot free with adding 2 spoonfuls of Rosewater for the scent and for softening the skin and 2 tablespoons full of milk to moisturize this skin surface.

After 30 minutes, you would wash off this paste, after rubbing it off with warm water. The final washing would be in cold water in the summer and warm water in the winter.

Along with this, they boosted up their intake of 3 parts of carrots, 2 parts of tomatoes, and one part of beetroot juice, mixed together and drank half a glass of this mixture for the next 15 – 20 days. This got rid of all the toxins, wrinkles, skin ailments, blemishes, and pimples. You could also take carrot juice and orange juice, if you lived in an area, where there were no tomatoes, especially in the ancient worlds.

This juice was taken at 3 – 4 o'clock in the afternoon. You did not eat or drink anything for an hour after/before taking this juice. The minimum time for this particular treatment was 20 days, and if you want to gain full healing benefits from it, continue it for 2 months for a permanent cure.

Natural Skin Lightening and Anti-Tanning Methods

Excessive exposure to the sun is going to have a harmful effect as well as cause harmful sunburn by exposing the skin to direct sunlight.

Traditionally, the best skin lightening agent was lemon juice in water. Ancient beauties put the juice of 2 fresh lemons in a bucket full of cold water and had a bath every day in the summer with this perfumed bath. After that, they rubbed the skin of the lemon, all over their bodies. This helped in the bleaching of the skin. In the winter, you could use warm water for your bath. This is also excellent for opening up the pores and lightening the skin tone.

Let me tell you how I do this treatment on myself. I love boiling hot showers – which is terribly dehydrating and drying for a skin, so I just squeeze a lemon into a mug full of warm water.

Remember that loofah glove we saw in the loofah section? After I have done my mud bath treatment with fuller's earth, mixed with a little bit of milk and chickpea flour, and got rid of all the dust and grime, I broil myself a little bit under the shower to get rid of the first installment of the bath.

After that, I get out of the shower, sit down on the side of the bathtub, dip my gloved palm into the lemon juice mixture, and smooth the solution, all over my face and body, not neglecting elbows, legs, feet, toes, and the back of my neck. This dipping and polishing is going to be thorough with absolutely not an inch overlooked or neglected.

This is going to give my whole skin, the lemon treatment, and keep it disease-free. Also, if there is any possibility of any infection going anywhere, this lemon water is going to get rid of potential warts and possible skin and fungal infections.

When I was living in tropical lands as a child, where my friends were genetically of a darker and dusky complexion, their mothers used a traditional way in order to lighten the complexion in the absence of lemons.

They used tamarind. This is a native fruit and you are going to use the brown and ripe pulp by putting 3 lumps into 250 g of water for about 2 hours until the pulp grew soft and mushy like papier-mâché.

This was made into chutney with pulp and water and applied all over your skin. This was allowed to dry on for 15 to 20 minutes and then you had your bath. This bleached the skin within 15 to 20 days, and the skin tone grew fairer as long as you kept up the treatment.

Incidentally, I envied them their genetically inherited smooth, attractive, blemish free and dusky complexions, because they did not have to bother about sunburn, suntan, and other blemishes which showed up so quickly on fairer complexions. On the other hand, they would moan that they wanted a complexion like mine. So nice and white, naa.

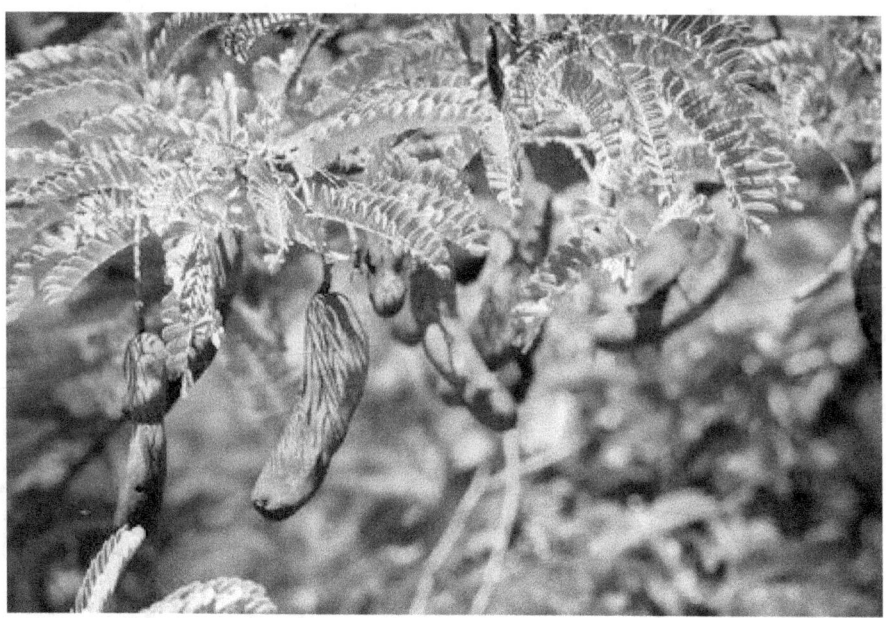

A Tamarind Tree

So, from childhood, I was psychologically geared to believe that anything fairer was immediately desirable. Especially when it was parents of my friends doing the praising of the complexions while patting the cheeks of my brother and I and sighing enviously and deeply.

Ah, well, the grass is always greener and always will be.

This was done in the summer, for up to 3 – 4 weeks at least twice a week.

You would also want to increase your intake of raisins, grapes, sultanas, carrots, milk, and other raw fruit and vegetables into your diet.

The idea of taking a cup full of tea or coffee first thing in the morning, has become such a major part of human lifestyle, that one immediately adds to the caffeine intake every day without even bothering at the long-term repercussions.

I remember a couple of my colleagues who could not manage to make any sort of decision or take on any responsible task without yelling for coffee. They were pure coffee addicts and I was sure that coffee deprivation would be as painful as nicotine deprivation for a smoker for them.

People do not seem to notice that this addiction to caffeine is almost as bad as an addiction to tobacco.

That is why am going to tell you the best way in which you can get rid of this craving for caffeine or tannin first thing in the morning.

You are going to take a copper utensil. Look for a pure copper jug, or glass, online. I normally put a liter of water in my copper jug overnight, and drink it poured into my copper glass, first thing in the morning.

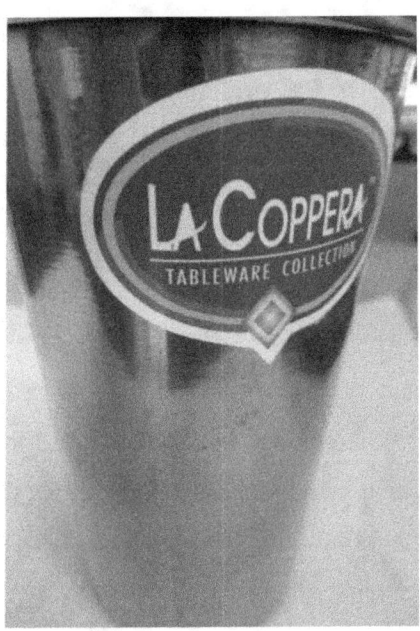

In ancient times, this copper water was drunk to get rid of any sort of mineral deficiency in the body, clear the system of toxins, clean the blood, as well as the skin.

How effective do I find it, you may ask. Well, I do not suffer from constipation, skin ailments, have plenty of energy, have never suffered from dehydration, and best of all, I am drinking lots of water, first thing in the morning, which was allowed to soak up minerals overnight and that means no copper deficiency. That means a cleared system within half an hour of waking up and drinking this copper water.

You may want to substitute a glass full of milk or a glass full of warm water and lemon and honey instead of tea and coffee. Try it out as an alternative. The ancients lived long and healthy, on these natural drinks.

Also, the ancients ate these natural fruits and vegetables along with milk, buttermilk, butter, and other natural milk products in their diet, in large quantity. These were apples, grapes, lemons, pomegranates, oranges, carrots, beet roots, radishes, radish leaves, spinach, fenugreek, almonds, and aniseed, coconut, and rock candy. This would keep you eternally young and youthful looking.

Nowadays, I enjoy a natural salad of radish, carrots, onions, tomatoes, beet roots, with spinach soup, as a tasty way to keep healthy and have a young looking and healthy skin.

Some years ago I saw a really beautiful old lady doing a traditional treatment to keep her skin looking young and blemish free. She took 4 almonds and soaked them in the morning. At bedtime, she took some fresh milk and crushed the almonds into them. This was her almond milk paste as smooth as butter.

She applied this all over her face, neck, and hands and went off to sleep and she had the softest, smoothest and loveliest apple cheeked and wrinkle free pale complexioned skin of any 85-year-old I had ever seen. The next morning she washed this almond milk first thing in the morning with cold water. I am hundred percent certain that the almond oil in the almond milk kept her skin youthful looking and well moisturized, as well as the added milk.

She told me that she had had a very hard life and nobody in their village could afford any expensive skin cream. But healthy fruit and vegetables, milk, and almonds they had in plenty in their area. So they did what their ancestors did, lived constructive and tension free lives bringing up their kids and grandkids, sang, laughed, talked, taught, prayed, and gave sincere thanks for all the days given to them.

I think this is the best lifestyle of which anybody could think. You can also use this almond milk solution one hour before you have a bath, if you do not want to apply it on your face at night and go to sleep with this paste on your skin which needs to breathe at night.

Also, she told me that nobody knew anything about soaps except Lifebuoy in her area! Many people could not afford it because times were hard in the Twenties and Thirties after the Great War. So naturally, they did not bother about using any sort of soap as a bathing cleanser, but instead used a paste of chickpea flour with a little bit of milk to clean the skin, as was done by her ancestors for millenniums.

Good sense.

Getting Rid of Wrinkles

The best natural way to get rid of wrinkles is just taking half a spoonful of fresh milk cream in which you have added 4 – 5 drops of lemon juice. Incidentally, I slathered this all over my face, before I began work on this book. So I am allowing the lemon to do its work while I am doing my routine work. That means moisturizing the skin, bleaching it, and getting rid of any possible blemishes. All at the same time.

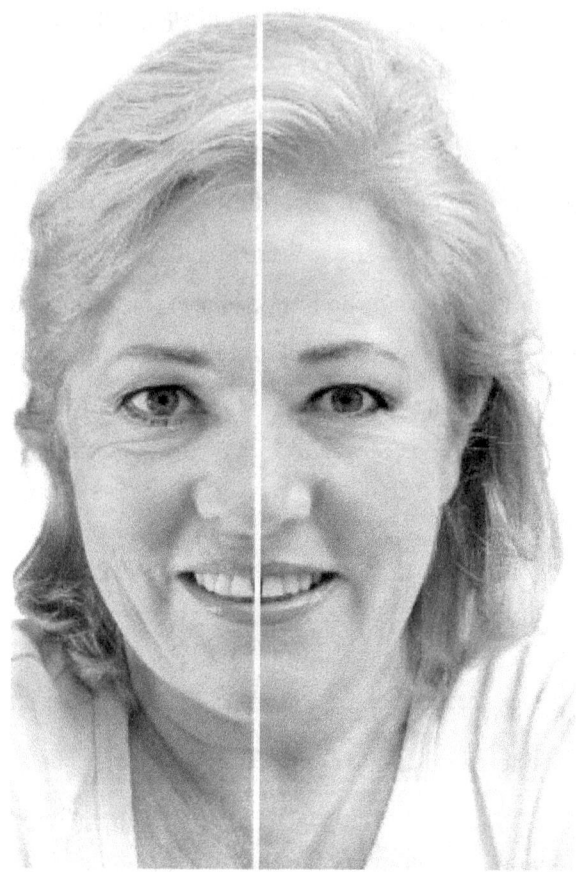

The atmosphere being a little bit cold, rainy, and blustery outside, it is going to take a little while for the cream and the lemon to get absorbed. But well, no wrinkles, no blemishes, also winter dullness and dry skin disappearing.

If you want to get rid of wrinkles, you are going to rub this all over your skin, before you go to sleep, especially in the areas where there are wrinkles. For this, first of all, you are going to wash your face with lukewarm water, and rub your face to get the circulation going with a rough towel.

After that you are going to rub lemon and cream all over your skin until all the cream is absorbed in the skin.

I am not doing any rubbing because I am just using it as a tonic instead of a wrinkle remover. When you do the rubbing, you are moisturizing your skin. If you do not want to keep it on overnight, you can take a bath, after half an hour.

Do this regularly for 15 – 20 days, once a day, and forget about wrinkles forever.

Also, you are not going to suffer from age spots, sunspots, and even liver spots on your face, neck, and hands.

When I was swapping this recipe with one of my Italian friends, she immediately shouted me down that everybody in her land knew all about it for centuries, and they did a massage of olive oil, after they took their bath. So I think you may want to do a little bit of massaging the skin with olive oil, to keep it soft and fragrant and beautiful looking.

An Oil Polish

When you are massaging your face with oil, remember that it should be squeaky clean. You are going to use 3 fingers to massaging the opposite direction of the wrinkles with warm olive oil. On your forehead, you are going to do the massaging with both of your palms in the upward direction. You are also going to take your fingers towards your temples and cheekbones. On your cheeks, you are going to do a soft circular motion. The rest of the skin on your face is going to be massaged towards your forehead, and ears. When you are massaging your cheeks, you are going to start from your chin region towards your ears.

For your chin, you are going to massage on the right and left side of your jawbone. When you are wiping your mouth, you start from beneath the chin towards your temple.

Also, if you have wrinkles on your hands, you are going to do the massaging towards the direction of your heart on your fingers with this milk and lemon juice solution. Followed by olive oil.

Papaya Treatment

I also found that pieces of papaya were extremely effective when the pulp was applied on the face. When it was dry, it was rubbed off with warm water and you took your shower. This was excellent for getting rid of wrinkles, moisturizing your face, and even body if you had plenty of papayas, blemishes, and dirt.

I was a baby when I lived in the land of plenty of papayas in a tropical paradise. That is when father kept trying to persuade us that the papayas gathered from the garden were really delicious. My younger brother and I were fed up with papayas, literally and figuratively. So we surreptitiously fed our portions to our pet mutt – after taking one spoonful – who loved them and thus was the healthiest mutt in the area.

In fact, this is the best pulp to get rid of wrinkles in the neck area. You are going to apply it all over your neck 5 minutes before you take your shower. This gets rid of all the dirt, grime, wrinkles, tan on the skin, and folds in the neck.

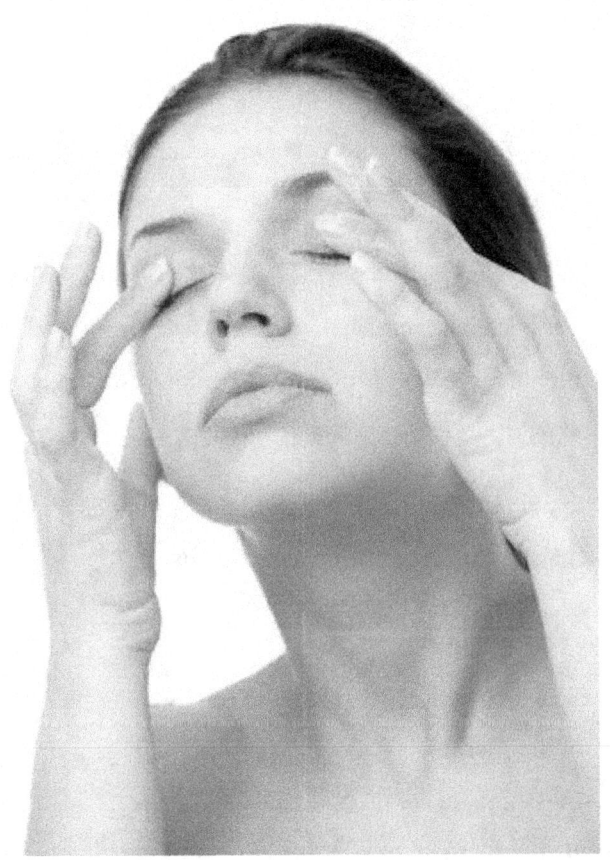

The wrinkles by the corners of the eyes can be gotten rid of with small pieces of cucumber placed in that area. You can also place them on your forehead, lie down on the carpet/bed and relax your body for the next 20 minutes. Do this for 2 weeks, and then tell me where your wrinkles went.

In ancient times, women getting ready to sleep and giving their kitchen a last cleaning sweep mixed a little bit of flour in some milk cream and applied it all over their faces. By the time the kitchen was quite clean, it was time for them to get rid of the grime by rubbing off the milk and flour paste with their fingers and palms.

After that, they washed their face with cold water and thus they never suffered from any wrinkles on their cheeks, around their eyes and black circles around their eyes ever. Also, no age spots and blemishes.

If you had wrinkles on your cheeks, all you had to do was rub the affected area with lemon juice, and massage your skin with this lemon juice with the help of the lemon peel. After 20 minutes, you could wash your face with cold water and pat it dry.

The rest of the wrinkles on the skin could be discouraged and prevented with just one glass of fresh carrot juice every day.

Thick Brows and Eyelashes

About a decade ago, a makeup artist to the stars was invited to our aviation training school in order to give the management and the trainee students lessons on professional makeup. Naturally, we managers and faculty members went straight there to pick up some tips, whether we used them or not.

Those were the days when eyebrows were sternly plucked and shaped, but I liked mine unplucked, because according to the art of physiognomy and face reading – an amusing Chinese tradition, my natural eyebrows were shaped in a "good spiritual way," just like that of John Lennon's! As I admired that gent's talent immensely, this worked fine with me.

I liked them thick and unshaped and untouched. So did he. He loved them. He really really did.[3] He had not seen unplucked eyebrows in a female for the last 25 years, he really really did not.

So he told us that the best way in which you could get really thick eyelashes and eyebrows was simple castor oil, applied every night before you went to sleep on your eyebrows and eyelashes. You did this 2 or 3 times a week. But I wanted thicker eyelashes and tried this treatment every night, along with wiping my eyebrows with my fingers of one hand, when applying oil on my scalp at the same time.

This is the best way in which you can get really thick eyebrows and eyelashes within a couple of months or even sooner, depending on the state of your health.

Preventing Chapped Lips

This is a rather amusing traditional remedy, which my grandmother did for us children, when we were kids. In winter, she made sure that after we had had our hot showers prior to going to sleep, she used to dip a finger in warm clarified butter and rotate it in our button-holes in winter. This navel tickling made us giggle a lot. Especially after which, she would listen to our prayers, and then we were kissed on our fore-heads, and tucked into sleep with blessings.

---

[3] Later on I found out he was Gay. Also, this was his natural way of speaking, so I did not find that effusive public appreciation embarrassing. Especially with all my colleagues, fluttering their hands and saying *really, really nice brows* whenever they were in a nasty mood and wanted to see me squirm.

Incidentally, I gave him a term, which he really really loved, and incorporated in all his future talks about makeup. "Black circles around the eyes which made one look like a panda."

Surprisingly enough, we never suffered from chapped lips and other dry skin problems, because according to her, this was the way in which skin would never dry anywhere when we were asleep.

I remember once when dad had to put us to sleep because she was busy on something else. We were not going to go to sleep, without the kiss, and he really did not know how the prayer routine went. Oh no not we. It was spring, and we were full of energy. In fact, this was a good opportunity for us to tell him that we absolutely could not go to sleep because we were not sleepy.

"Nonsense," he said, "how can you say you are not sleepy, when I can see the little sleep fairy sitting right there on your noses, – Tapping our noses – just close your eyes so that she can sit on your eyelashes. She knows you are tired little babies and she is also tired and she wants to go to sleep – tapping our eyelashes –. So good night!" And he snapped off the lights and left us. We were asleep within 30 seconds. Parents knew all about child psychology at that time! Especially parents with imagination.

Dark Elbows

Elbows are normally neglected, because one forgets to scrub them, when in the shower. So if you find your elbows darker than your normal arm color tone, just cut a lemon into 2, and rub it all over your elbows with the help of the lemon peel and lemon juice. After 3 – 4 hours, you are going to find the grime ready to be removed. Scrub your elbows with a rough towel dipped in hot water. Do this regularly every day until your elbows are soft, smooth, and clean.

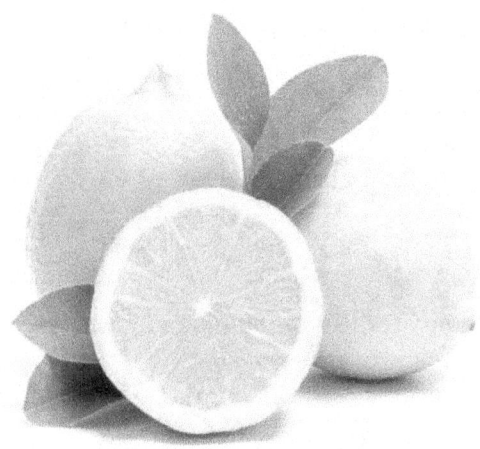

This treatment has to be done on your knees, ankles, soles of your feet, toes, fingers, and nails by rubbing them with pieces of lemon peel and lemon juice and leaving the juice on for half an hour when you are going to get rid of the dead cells with the help of the rubbing once again with the lemon peel. This would give your skin surface a squeaky clean and really smooth polish.

Believe it or not, half of the lemons I buy or pick from the garden for home consumption go into such activities, instead of being eaten!

Smoothing Rough Skin

If any portion of your body feels rough, chapped or thick, you can make it soft and smooth by rubbing lemon all over it at night, and going to sleep. This is going to make the skin soft and remove the thickness and rough texture.

Also, I found out that when I was doing this treatment with lemon peel, it removed the strong odor of garlic and onions, which may have clung to my hands during the cooking of the evening's meal. Also, it kept my hands soft, clean, dirt-free, and younger looking and absolutely no dishwasher hands.

Getting Rid of Corns

When corn caps were not in existence, corns were removed by rubbing the corns morning, and night with castor oil for a few minutes. The corns fell off within 2 – 3 weeks.

Getting Rid of Warts and Moles.

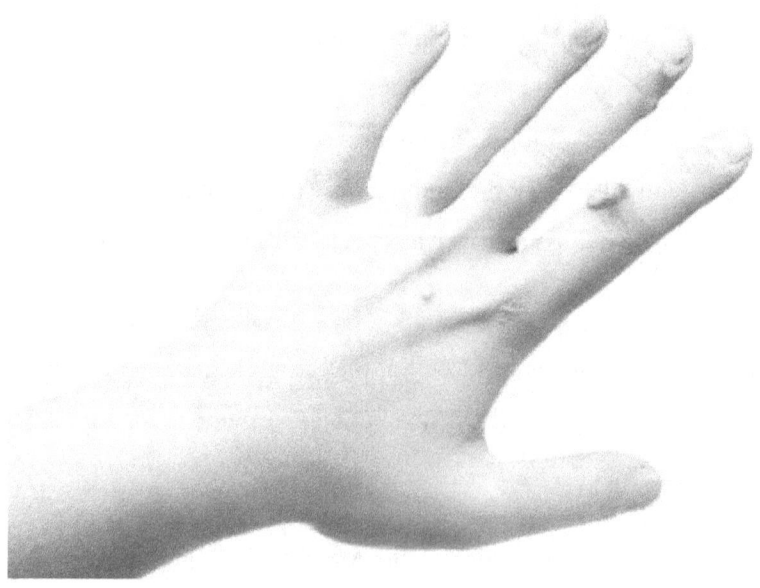

Calcium hydroxide – also known as pickling lime – food grade – is going to be used the traditional way to get rid of warts. Just take a little bit of ginger and peel it in the shape of a lead pencil point. Now dip it into one wheat grain sized amount powder of pickling lime. Rub it all over your wart so that ginger juice mixed with calcium hydroxide is rubbed all over the wart slowly.

The skin is going to swell up a little because of the action of the calcium hydroxide. But you are soon going to find the wart falling off without any scar or mark.

You can also apply castor oil on your warts every day, until the warts fall off. This is a long-term treatment because warts are viruses and you are disturbing them with the castor oil. Castor oil is also excellent to get rid of spots, liver spots, and moles on parts of your body, with a massage done 2 – 3 times a day. This is going to loosen the hold the wart has in the epidermis of the skin and it is going to drop and fall off without leaving an unsightly scar.

Healthy Nails

Many people are annoyed because their nails are not healthy and crack easily. Some of them looked disfigured.

You can get healthy nails easily by just dipping a wad of cotton into some lemon juice or just rub a little bit of lemon peel all over your nails. Wash your hands after some time. Do this for a number of days until you find your nails growing strong and healthy looking.

You can also use warm olive oil on your nails and massage them slowly and gently. This is excellent to strengthen weak nails.

Let me tell you something amusing here. Dip your hands in Dishwashing soap suds and warm water for 5 minutes and dry them before you try the olive oil treatment. The soap suds and warm water seemed to have a positive effect in helping in the growth of the nails.

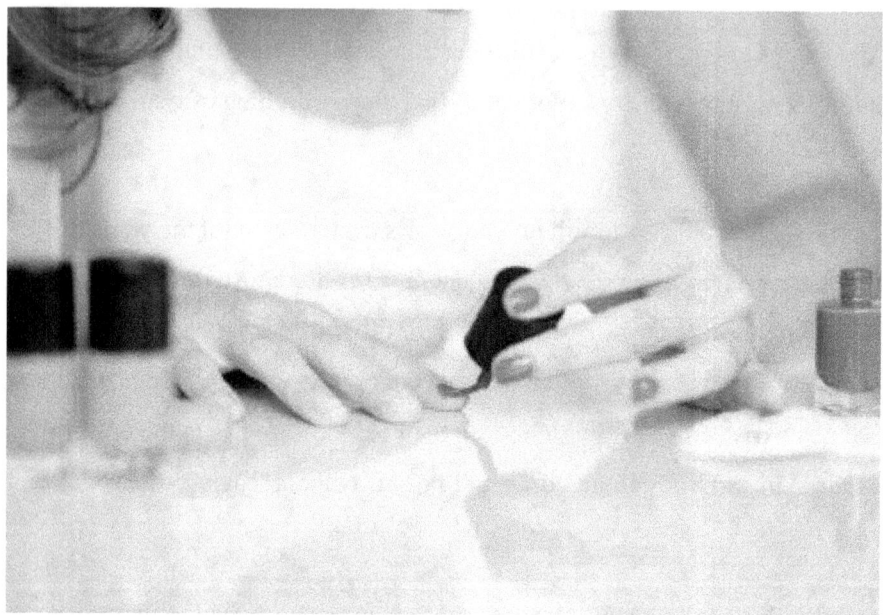

Cracked nails and chipped nails can be made healthy by just dipping them in warm mustard oil or olive oil for 10 minutes. After that, rub the nails so that the blood circulation in that area is done properly. Try this for a week, to strengthen your nails.

Boost up your calcium intake in the form of eggs and milk. This is going to encourage your nails to grow. You could also encourage them to grow in a more physical manner by dipping them for 5 minutes in warm water in which you have put in some lemon juice. Leave them like that for 5 minutes, rubbing your fingers and nails slowly. After that, dip them immediately in cold water. This is going to set the nails growing while keeping them healthy and soft.

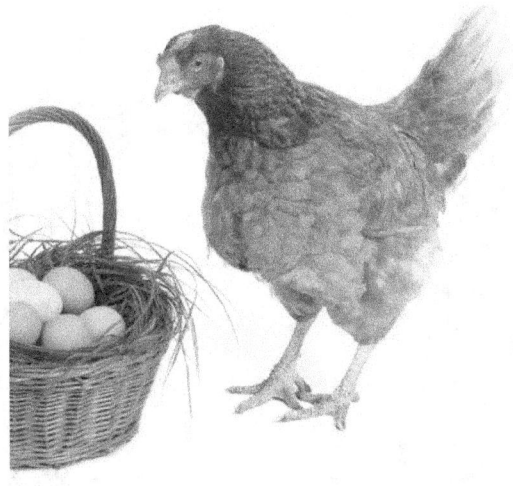

Lots of eggs means healthy nails, skin, and healthy hair

If you are suffering from anemia, there is a chance that this is the reason why your nails are not growing so well. For this, you are going to take 15 to 25 raisins soaked overnight in a cup of water and the water drunk and the raisins chewed first thing in the morning.

Do this anywhere between 15 – 25 days. This is going to get rid of any potential anemia problems by supplying the iron deficiency. So apart from your healthy nails, you are going to have a healthy glow to your skin and hair as well as the palms of your hands.

Conclusion

This book has told you a lot of traditional body care methods which have been used all over the world to keep your skin healthy, younger looking, and rejuvenated.

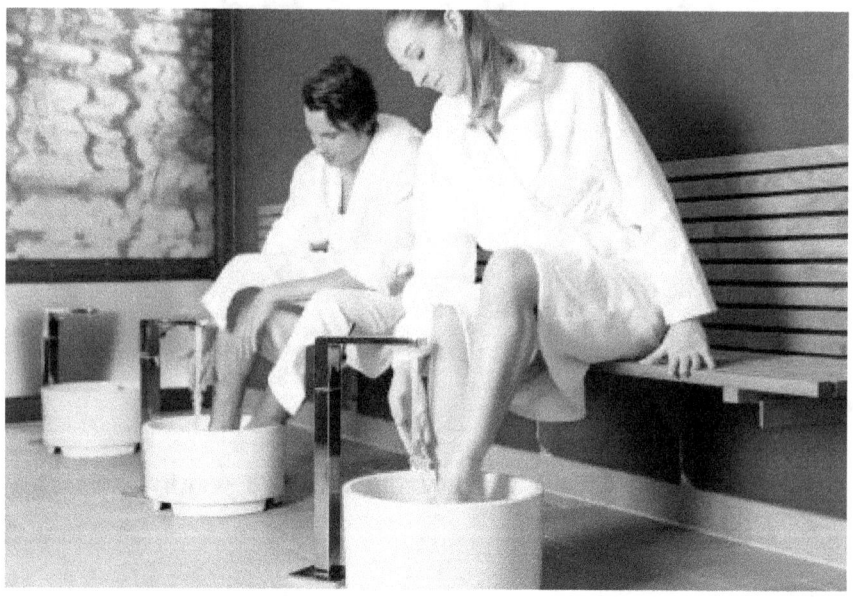

Here are some other tips, which can keep the rest of you healthy. Try massaging the soles of your feet with your own palms. This increases and improves your vision while relaxing you. It also helps improve the circulation throughout your body and prevents age-related ailments. This is because there are plenty of pressure points in the bottom of the feet, especially the sole area that are related to other parts of the body and heal them, naturally.

Also, you are not going to suffer from cramps ever in your hands and feet. Do this once or twice a week, for a healthy person before going to sleep. He is going to remain healthy throughout his life. He is also never going to suffer from heart ailments, paralysis, blood pressure, diabetes, sciatica, cervical spondylitis, gout, problems in your spinal cord, and lungs. Do this regularly, and you are going to get rid of all the toxins in your body naturally. This is going to strengthen the natural immune system of your body.

So that means you are going to get rid of simple or chronic infections and diseases permanently and naturally.

In ancient times, this massage was done by a person with the palms of his hands and a little warm clarified butter on the soles of his feet. At that time, it was believed that the pressure points in the hands had their direct counterparts in pressure points in your head. Massaging the soles' pressure points was directly related to your heart. So you would never suffer from heart attacks or heart related problems.

So keep your sole and heels well massaged and you are going to find yourselves suffering from no physical head and heart problems including stress, tension, headache, and brain related diseases.

So keep healthy the natural way, Live Long and Prosper!

Author Bio

Dueep Jyot Singh is a Management and IT Professional who managed to gather Postgraduate qualifications in Management and English and Degrees in Science, French and Education while pursuing different enjoyable career options like being an hospital administrator, IT,SEO and HRD Database Manager/ trainer, movie , radio and TV scriptwriter, theatre artiste and public speaker, lecturer in French, Marketing and Advertising, ex-Editor of Hearts On Fire (now known as Solstice) Books Missouri USA, advice columnist and cartoonist, publisher and Aviation School trainer, ex-moderator on Medico.in, banker, student councilor ,travelogue writer … among other things!

One fine morning, she decided that she had enough of killing herself by Degrees and went back to her first love -- writing. It's more enjoyable! She already has 48 published academic and 14 fiction- in- different- genre books under her belt.

When she is not designing websites or making Graphic design illustrations for clients , she is browsing through old bookshops hunting for treasures, of which she has an enviable collection – including R.L. Stevenson, O.Henry, Dornford Yates, Maurice Walsh, De Maupassant, Victor Hugo, Sapper, C.N. Williamson, "Bartimeus" and the crown of her collection- Dickens "The Old Curiosity Shop," and "Martin Chuzzlewit" and so on… Just call her "Renaissance Woman" - collecting herbal remedies, acting like Universal Helping Hand/Agony Aunt, or escaping to her dear mountains for a bit of exploring, collecting herbs and plants, and trekking.

Check out some of the other JD-Biz Publishing books

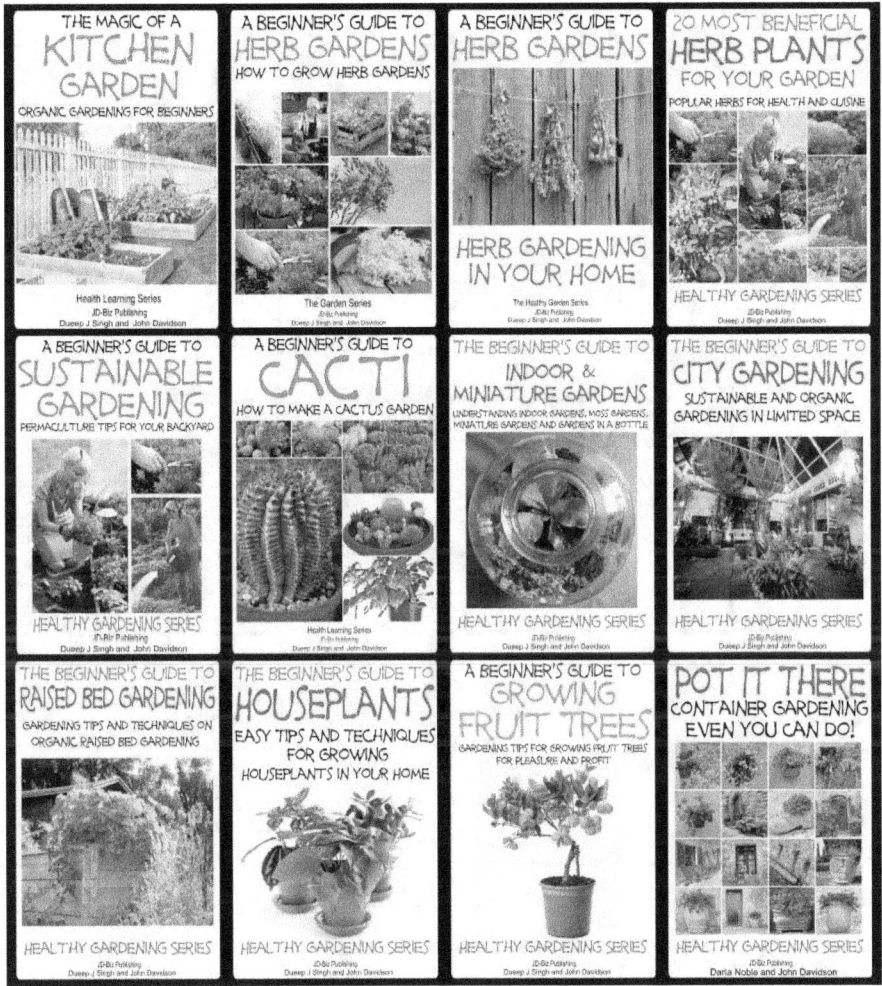

THE MAGIC OF GOOSEBERRIES FOR HEALTH AND BEAUTY — Natural Remedy Series

THE MAGIC OF YOGURT FOR COOKING AND BEAUTY — Natural Remedy Series

THE MAGIC OF LEMONS USING LEMONS FOR HEALTH AND BEAUTY — Natural Remedy Series

THE MAGIC OF CHILLIES FOR COOKING AND HEALING — Natural Remedy Series

THE MAGIC OF ONIONS ONIONS IN CUISINE TO CURE AND TO HEAL — Natural Remedy Series

THE MAGIC OF RADISHES TO CURE AND TO HEAL — Natural Remedy Series

THE MAGIC OF CARROTS TO CURE AND TO HEAL — Natural Remedy Series

THE HEALTH BENEFITS OF OREGANO FOR COOKING AND HEALTH — Natural Remedy Series

The Magic Of MARIGOLDS Marigolds for Health And Beauty — Natural Remedy Series

THE HEALTH BENEFITS OF CINNAMON — Natural Remedy Series

THE MAGIC OF COCONUTS FOR COOKING & HEALTH — Health Learning Series

THE MAGIC OF CLOVES FOR HEALING AND COOKING — Health Learning Series

THE MAGIC OF ASAFETIDA FOR COOKING AND HEALING — Health Learning Series

THE MAGIC OF NEEM MARGOSA TO HEAL — Natural Remedy Series

THE MAGIC OF SALT TO HEAL AND FOR BEAUTY — Natural Remedy Series

THE MAGIC OF POMEGRANATES FOR HEALTH AND BEAUTY — Natural Remedy Series

THE MAGIC OF DRY FRUIT AND SPICES REMEDIES AND RECIPES — Natural Remedy Series

THE HEALTH BENEFITS OF TURMERIC CURCUMIN FOR COOKING AND HEALTH — Natural Remedy Series

THE MAGIC OF ALOE VERA — Natural Remedy Series

THE MAGIC OF VEGETABLES ANCIENT HEALING REMEDIES AND TIPS — Natural Remedy Series

THE HEALTH BENEFITS OF ROSEMARY FOR COOKING AND HEALTH — Natural Remedy Series

THE MAGIC OF PEPPER & PEPPERCORNS FOR COOKING & HEALING — Natural Remedy Series

THE MAGIC OF MILK, BUTTER AND CHEESE FOR COOKING & HEALING — Natural Remedy Series

THE MAGIC OF CARDAMOMS FOR COOKING AND HEALTH — Health Learning Series

THE HEALTH BENEFITS OF BLACK CUMIN FOR COOKING AND HEALTH — Natural Remedy Series

THE MAGIC OF BASIL-TULSI TO HEAL NATURALLY — Health Learning Series

THE MAGIC OF SPICES FOR HEALTH AND CUISINE — Natural Remedy Series

THE MAGIC OF ROSES FOR COOKING AND BEAUTY — Natural Remedy Series

The Miraculous Healing Powers of GINGER — Natural Remedy Series BEST

The Miracle of HONEY — Natural Remedy Series BEST

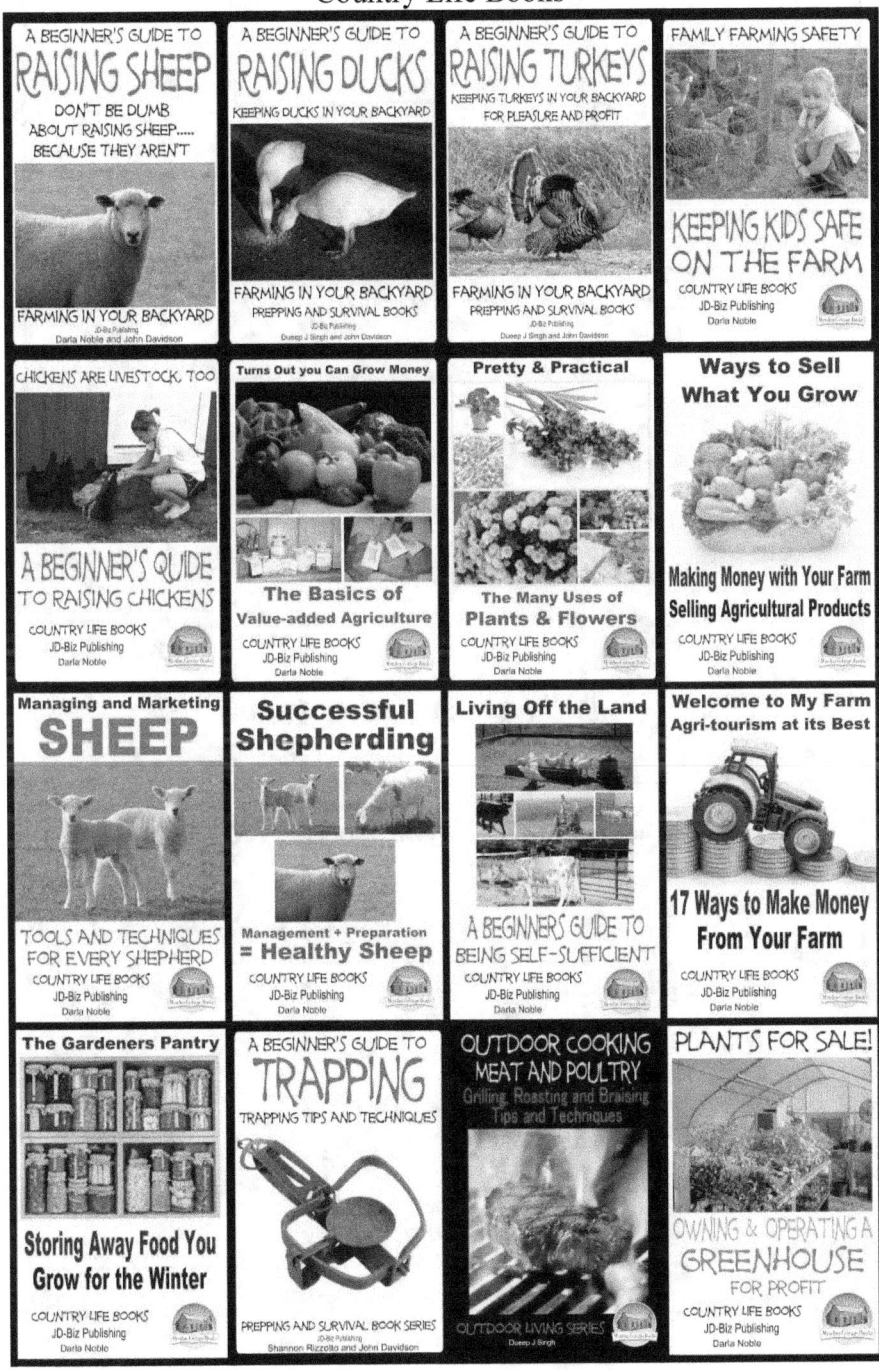

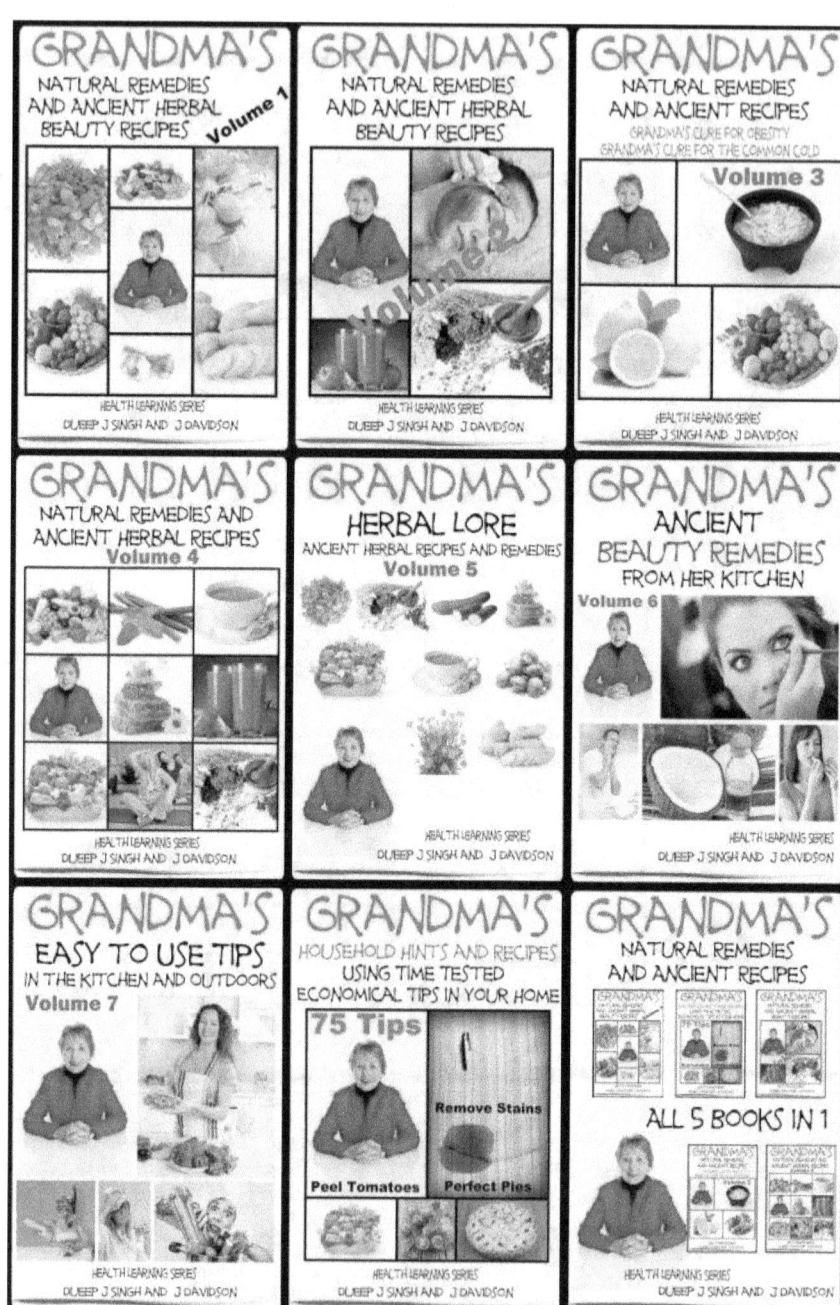

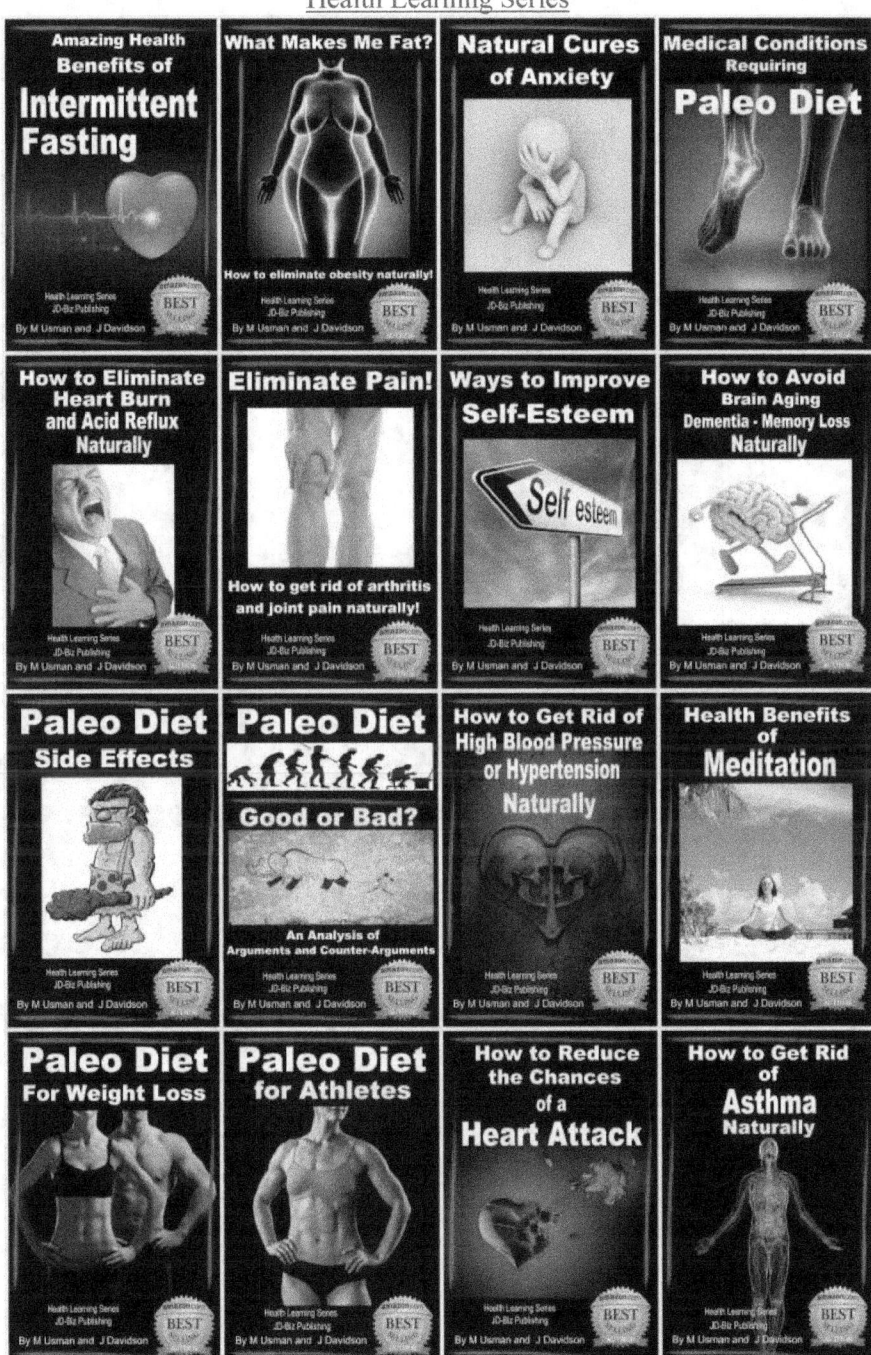

<u>Amazing Animal Book Series</u>

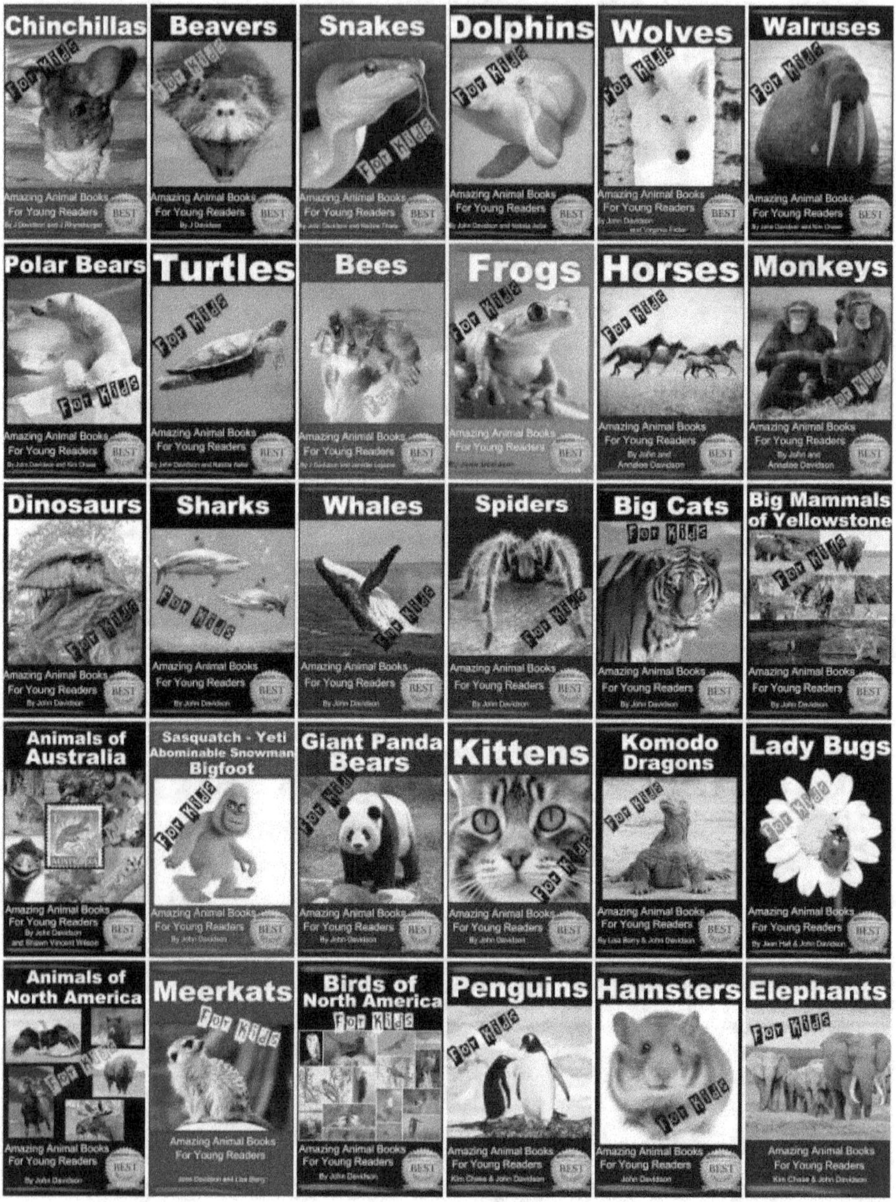

Learn To Draw Series

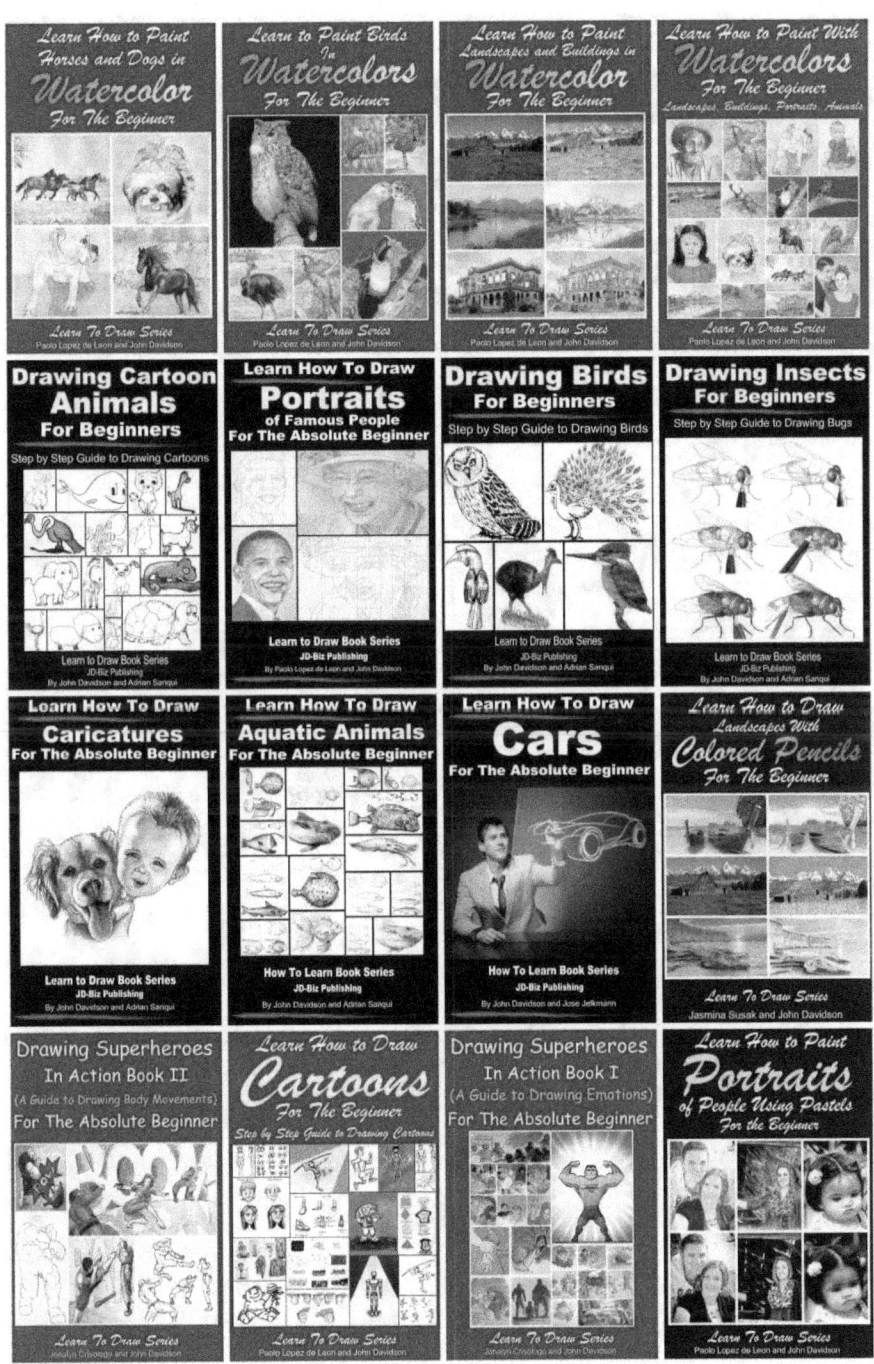

How to Build and Plan Books

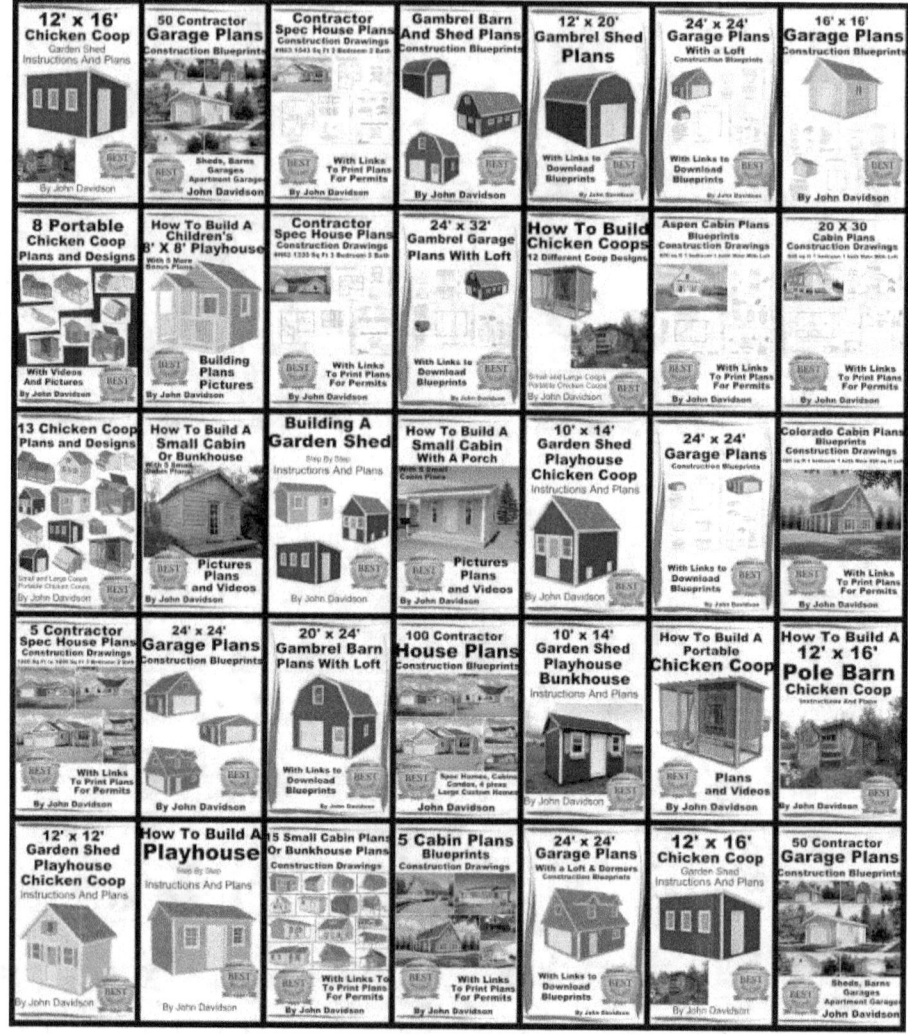

Entrepreneur Book Series

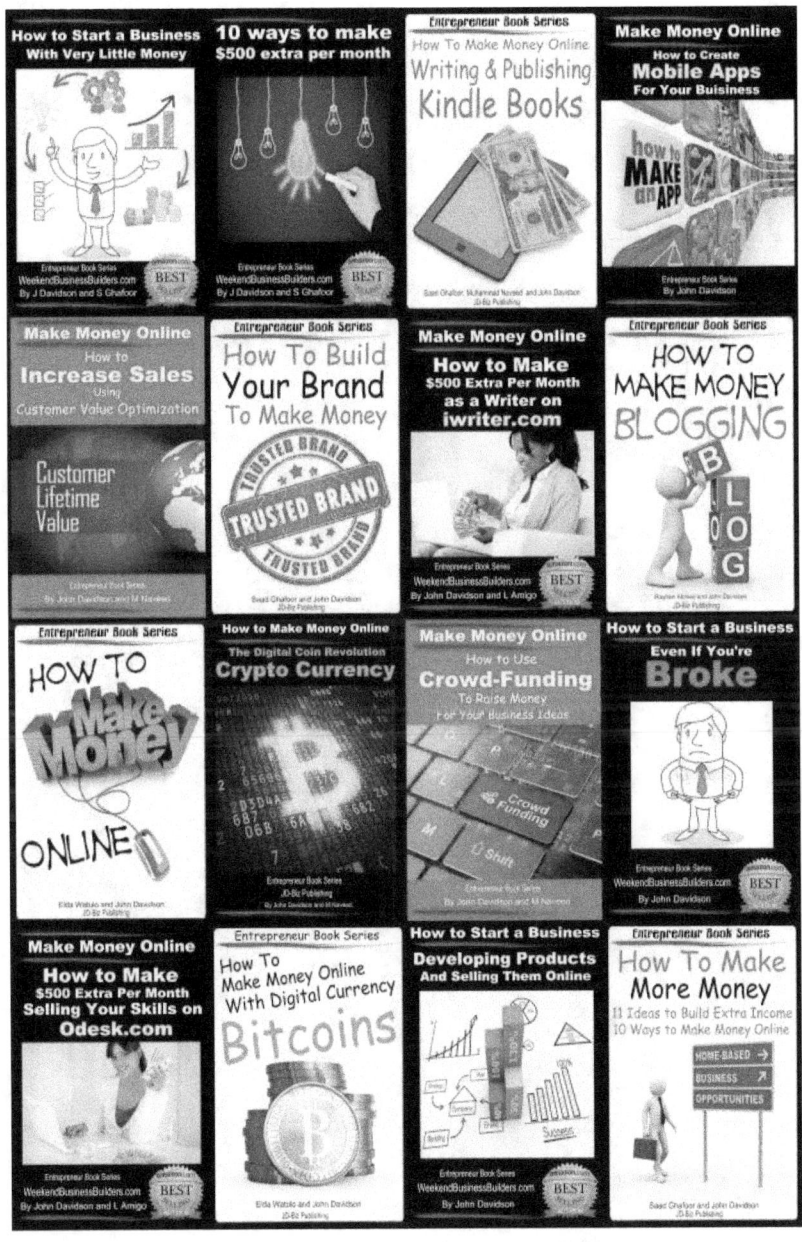

Our books are available at

1. Amazon.com

2. Barnes and Noble

3. Itunes

4. Kobo

5. Smashwords

6. Google Play Books

Download Free Books!

http://MendonCottageBooks.com

Publisher

JD-BIZ PUBLISHING

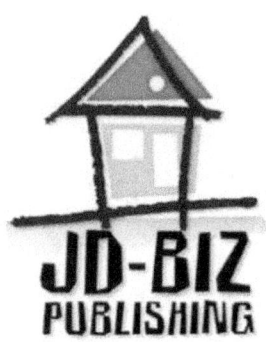

JD-Biz Corp

P O Box 374

Mendon, Utah 84325

http://www.jd-biz.com/

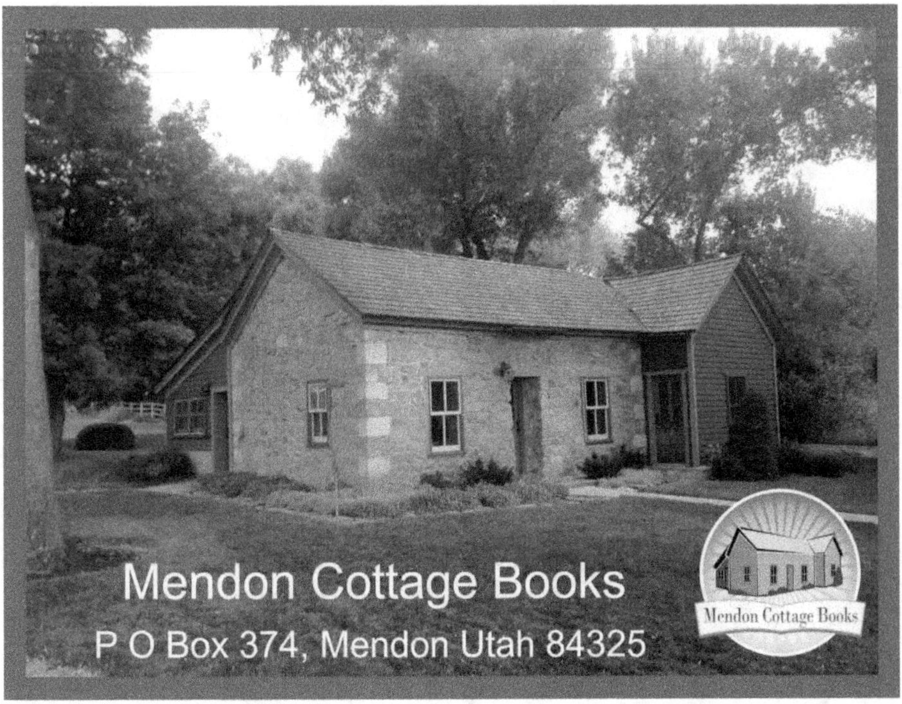

Mendon Cottage Books
P O Box 374, Mendon Utah 84325
Mendon Cottage Books

www.ingramcontent.com/pod-product-compliance
Lightning Source LLC
Chambersburg PA
CBHW071248280526
45788CB00004B/1624